THE
MAGICAL
SECRETS OF
HEALING

Ancient Remedies and Diet Hacks with Mystical Age Reversing Properties

by

James Belgiovine

Table of Contents

The following eBook is reproduced below with the goal of providing information that is as accurate and reliable as possible. Regardless, purchasing this eBook can be seen as consent to the fact that both the publisher and the author of this book are in no way experts on the topics discussed within and that any recommendations or suggestions that are made herein are for entertainment purposes only. Professionals should be consulted as needed prior to undertaking any of the action endorsed herein.

This declaration is deemed fair and valid by both the American Bar Association and the Committee of Publishers Association and is legally binding throughout the United States.

Furthermore, the transmission, duplication or reproduction of any of the following work including specific information will be considered an illegal act irrespective of if it is done electronically or in print. This extends to creating a secondary or tertiary copy of the work or a recorded copy and is only allowed with express written consent from the Publisher. All additional right reserved.

The information in the following pages is broadly considered to be a truthful and accurate account of facts, and as such any inattention, use or misuse of the information in question by the reader will render any resulting actions solely under their purview. There are no scenarios in which the publisher or the original author of this work can be in any fashion deemed liable for any hardship or damages that may befall them after undertaking information described herein.

Additionally, the information in the following pages is intended only for informational purposes and should thus be thought of as universal. As befitting its nature, it is presented without assurance regarding its prolonged validity or interim quality. Trademarks that are mentioned are done without written consent and can in no way be considered an endorsement from the trademark holder.

Introduction

The book you hold in your hands contains secrets from the ancient world to help you live healthily, heal from diseases, increase longevity, and ultimately find happiness. These secrets have been passed down from our ancient ancestors throughout the world—in ancient Greece and Rome, China, India, and even Egypt. Each civilization from the past contains important practices that can help you heal faster, enjoy better health, and live a longer life. While in our contemporary world, many people have forgotten these secrets, they continue to be preserved through writing. This book will lead you through simple, daily practices that will drastically improve your quality of life.

One of the biggest secrets of the past is that many ancient cultures approached healing and health as a holistic process. The great doctor and philosopher from ancient Greece, Hippocrates, taught that a healthy individual would have both a healthy mind and a healthy body. The ancients also knew that the best way to heal ourselves was to rely on the power in our own bodies. Hippocrates taught, "Natural forces within us are the true healers of diseases." Ancient Indian and Chinese medical texts also teach us that there should be harmony between the mind and the body to attain optimal health. Without a healthy relationship between the organ systems within our body, there is no way to enjoy a healthy life.

Because of this, many of the recommendations found in this book will help both your body and mind to heal and remain healthy.

The secrets found in this book are also simple. The philosophers and doctors of ancient cultures did not believe in complicated procedures, but in taking advantage of the simple things, we do every day to encourage better health. In this book, you will find secrets on how to use sleep, a practice that we do every day, to help your body naturally heal and maintain health. Eating and drinking are also another important part of our daily lives that will greatly affect overall health. This book also contains the ancient secrets of fasting and abstaining from certain foods, to help you live longer and enjoy a life free from disease. Finally, this book will teach you the ancient secrets of meditation and how to adopt this practice into your daily life.

Health should be widely available to everyone and should not require expensive or complicated procedures. By looking to the past, you will be able to greatly influence your future.

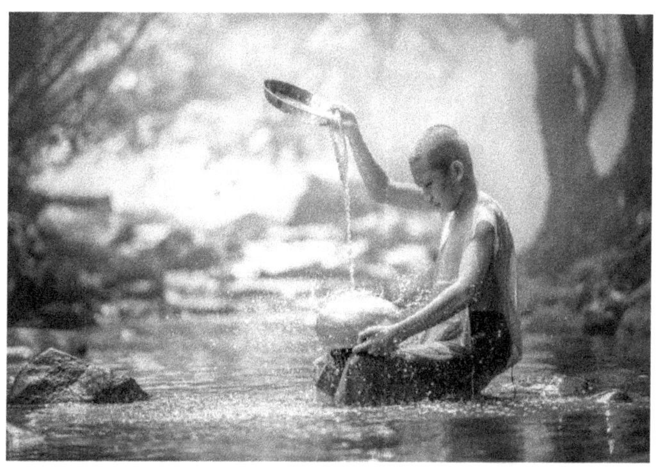

Chapter 1: Sleep

---

*"We are such stuff as
dreams are made on,
and our little life is
rounded with sleep."*

-William Shakespeare

Sleep is one of the most natural human functions that we perform, and one of the most important things we can do for our body's health. The average human will probably spend over twenty-five percent of their entire life sleeping. Even though we participate in this activity every day, we often overlook how important sleep can be for both the body and the mind. One of the best kept ancient secrets to improve your health, experience more energy, and feel an increased passion for life requires nothing more than examining your current approach to sleep.

Many ancient civilizations understood the importance of

sleep and created gods dedicated to this essential practice. In ancient Greece, for example, the people worshiped Hypnos, the winged god of sleep. Like most Greek gods, Hypnos has an extensive family, including his brother Thanatos, the god of death, and his children Morpheus, Phobetor, and Phantasos who watch over dreams.

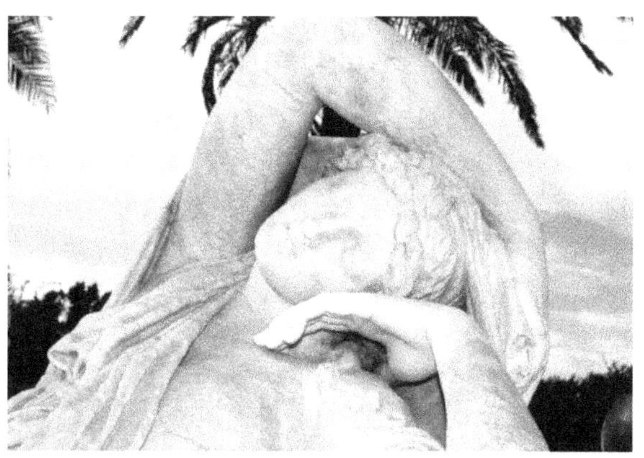

The god of sleep was so important to the Greeks that he played a major role in one of their fundamental origin stories—the Trojan War. In this legend, the Achaeans—ancient ancestors to the Greeks—fought against the Trojans; however, the Achaeans were losing. Hera wanted to help the Achaeans, but to do so, she needed Zeus to be distracted since he was supporting the Trojans at the time. Hera asked Hypnos to put Zeus to sleep so that he would be unable to bring aid to the Trojans. Hypnos agreed to the task, made Zeus fall asleep, and procured the help of Poseidon. With Hypnos's aid, the battle began to turn, and the Achaeans were able to win the war.

Other ancient cultures also have deities dedicated to sleep. In ancient Egypt, they worshiped

Tutu, their own god of sleep with a lion's body, man's head, and a serpent for a tail. Tutu was said to protect your dreams from nightmares and your waking hours from demons. Egyptians even expected to continue the practices of sleep in their afterlife and were often buried with beds, sheets, and neck rests used for sleeping.

Both the Greeks and the Egyptians also erected what is called sleep temples. In ancient Greece, instead of dedicating these temples to Hypnos, the god of sleep, these temples were built in honor of Asclepios, the god of medicine. The ancient Egyptians also built sleep temples that were unconnected with the patronage of any god. Instead, sleep temples were a place of healing and recovery, employing hypnosis techniques to encourage self-healing in the body. Such a history suggests that both the ancient Greeks and Egyptians understood the important connection between sleep and health.

You are probably familiar with the ancient proverb often attributed to Benjamin Franklin, who included it in his famous *Farmer's Almanacs*: "Early to bed and early to rise makes a man healthy, and wealthy, and wise." In addition to understanding the important connection between sleep and health, ancient civilizations also recognized the harms associated with oversleeping. Another member of Hypnos's family is Aergia, the goddess of laziness, indolence, and sloth. Ancient Greeks recognized that if they worshiped Hypnos too much, i.e., they overslept, they would be subject to the influence of Aergia. Likewise, in the eastern religion of Buddhism, Buddha taught the importance of enjoying a sleep in moderation. Since the followers of Buddha dedicated a lot of time to meditation, Buddha understood that oversleeping or sleeping during meditation hours could be a temptation. To prevent his followers from indulging in too much sleep, Buddha taught that the man or woman who wallows sleeping in a bed like a pig would be reborn again as a pig.

Unlike our ancient predecessors, in our modern world, we often ignore our body's signals that it needs sleep. And when we finally do give our body the sleep it craves, we tend to overindulge and sleep too much. Additionally, the sleep that we do get is often interrupted and lacks quality. In place of meditation and quiet, we try to drift off with bright phone screens in loud environments which disrupt our sleep patterns and prevent us from experience sleep fully. By constantly participating in sub-par sleep practices, we miss out on the many of the health benefits sleep has to offer and we also do not fully experience the sleep cycle.

The sleep cycle contains two phases called REM and NREM. REM stands for "rapid eye movement," and NREM means "non-rapid eye movement." To experience a good night's sleep, the body should cycle through both of these phases during the night. Many people believe that the REM phase is the only phase of sleep that matters, but the NREM phase is actually more important for our physical health. Luckily for us, the NREM phase occupies the majority of our sleeping time, over seventy-five percent, allowing our body ample time to experience many of sleep's health benefits during this phase. If you sleep the recommended seven or eight hours every night, only one hour is spent in REM sleep. The rest of the night, your body is working hard to repair itself and the major organ groups.

During the NREM phase, the body heals damaged cells and tissue, such as the heart and blood vessels, and repairs your skin. Those who frequently do not get enough sleep have a higher risk of heart disease, high blood pressure, and ultimately are at increased risk for strokes. But if you sleep enough, you can experience improved heart health and decrease your risk for many cardiovascular diseases. Furthermore, another benefit of getting enough sleep includes better kidney health and decreased inflammation throughout the body. While in the NREM sleep phase, the body also replenishes essential hormones, helping to rebalance the body's hormones in the process. For example, if you do not get enough sleep, your body's sensitivity to insulin (the hormone that helps your body process sugars and regulates your blood sugar levels) can decrease. This, in turn, leads to a higher risk for developing diabetes. But, if you do get the recommended seven or eight hours a night, then your body can resolve these issues all on its own. Other important hormones that lack of sleep can disrupt include collagen and the human growth hormone or HCG. These hormones are essential for healthy, firm, and younger-looking skin. In other words, getting a full night's sleep is a simple remedy for reversing the aging process!

Although the REM phase of sleep is not important for your physical health, there are many benefits to your mental health. The REM phase is the part of the sleep cycle when you dream. The mind's ability to create dreams allows it to sort through emotions, stresses, and even memories. Fully experiencing the REM phase can increase your problem-solving abilities and memory. It also prepares your brain to learn and develop new skills, which are essential elements of living life to the fullest.

Another important health benefit of getting enough sleep is controlling weight. In many medical studies, sleeping poorly is associated with weight gain and even obesity. One reason for this is that when people are sleep deprived, they usually have larger appetites and want to consume more calories. Hormone regulation is connected to this as well. When you do not sleep enough, your body produces more of the hormone ghrelin which encourages your appetite. Also, with a lack of sleep, the body decreases the production of the hormone leptin which suppresses your appetite. In other words, if you do not get enough sleep, your body will crave unhealthy foods, and you will want to overeat. However, if you do get enough sleep, your body will naturally want to eat less and stay more active—a win-win situation.

If you are not experiencing a good night's sleep, there are many ways that you can change your habits and improve the quality of sleep. One of the main ways to improve your sleep is to understand your body's natural cycles. Your body is more aware of itself than your mind is, oftentimes. It knows when it is sleepy, and it knows when it has had a full night's rest. If you go to bed when you are tired and wake up without the aid of an alarm, this can drastically improve your ability to enjoy sleeping. However, for many, this is an unrealistic expectation because people experience busy lives and strict schedules. If this is the case, you might have to set an earlier bedtime so that you can wake up without an alarm and still have time to prepare for your day. Another habit you should adopt is preparing for bed and waking up at the same time every day—even on weekends and holidays. By changing the times you go to bed and wake up, you can increase the quality of your sleep and improve your access to sleep's natural health benefits.

Your exposure to light can also influence the how well you are sleeping. Thousands of years ago, people did not have the luxury of electric lights. Their only light source came from the sun. Therefore, they had to wake up with the sun and stop their daily activities when the sunset. To replicate the patterns of our ancient ancestors, when you wake up it's essential that you expose yourself to bright sunlight. Also, if you spend more time outside during the day and increase your exposure to natural light, it will be easier to fall asleep when it becomes dark. At night, make sure your room is dark and cool. If you have to get up during the middle of the night, make sure you use low lights rather than the full, bright electric lights that will wake you up and disrupt your sleep patterns. Also, it's important that you avoid electronics near bedtime. This includes avoiding watching television, reading on back-lit devices, or staring at a bright phone screen. If you want to experience the health benefits of the ancients, then you must follow the practices of the ancients.

In addition to these simple habit changes, your sleep might also be disrupted because you lack the proper vitamins and minerals in your diet. One mineral that plays a critical and often unrecognized role in sleep is **Magnesium**. Low levels of Magnesium in the body have been connected to increased stress, more anxiety, and a harder time relaxing. And if you cannot relax and you feel stressed out, it will be harder for you to sleep well throughout the night.

Magnesium is abundant throughout the universe, including in our own earth's crust. This element develops mostly in aging stars and is dispelled to other solar systems from supernova blasts.

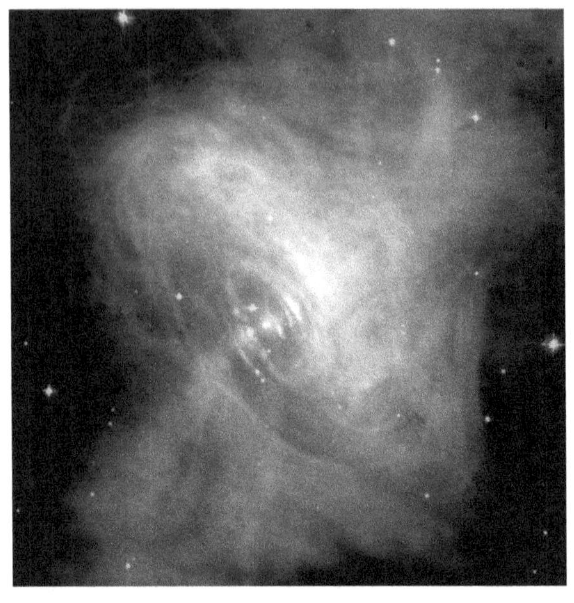

In ancient alchemy practices, Magnesium was an important element. When Magnesium is in its pure form and shaved into strips, it can easily catch on fire, and for this reason, it represented eternity and ascension. The name Magnesium comes from the district Magnesia in Thessaly—an ancient Greek civilization where this mineral was found in abundance. Although it appears that the ancient Greeks were unaware of Magnesium's ability to heal, they did use compounds of Magnesium to treat some diseases. For example, the ancient Greek doctor Hippocrates made many references to using magnetite—a Magnesium compound—in his healing practices. He recorded that ancient doctors used this mineral to stop and control excessive bleeding, cure burns, and reduce watering of the eyes of many adults.

While the Greeks may not have used Magnesium directly, the eastern medical traditions were more in tune with this metal's special powers. Traditional Chinese medicine has known about the healing properties of Magnesium for thousands of years. In this eastern medicine tradition, stable levels of Magnesium have been linked with the proper function of the gallbladder and liver, two organs which are directly associated with anxiety, nervousness, irritation, and anger. All of these behaviors associated with the gallbladder and liver are also the same behaviors that can negatively impact the quality of your sleep!

While Magnesium is found in many foods, almost half of all adults in the United States have difficulty absorbing Magnesium and do not get enough of this mineral from their diet. Women are especially at a high risk of

Magnesium deficiency. Taking a supplement helps many people increase their Magnesium levels and improve their quality of sleep. Many studies have been conducted on the connections between taking a Magnesium supplement and increased sleep quality. While this essential mineral will not increase the total time you sleep each night, it will help you fall asleep faster and make sure the time you spend in bed is spent actually sleeping rather than lying awake or thrashing about. In fact, many people who experience restlessness, especially in the form of restless leg syndrome, noted that they sleep better while taking a Magnesium supplement. This is because Magnesium can help control the brain's neurotransmitters, helping calm the nervous system down and relax the mind and body.

Magnesium works in conjunction with the brain to produce this relaxing effect. When Magnesium is ingested, it connects to the brain's gamma-aminobutyric acid receptors. These receptors are more commonly known as GABA receptors, and they can help reduce brain activity if the mind is overworked or overactive. If you lie awake at night experiencing racing thoughts or are constantly thinking about things that stress you out while trying to fall asleep, you make have low levels of gamma-aminobutyric acid.

While some medical traditions have been aware of the benefits of Magnesium for thousands of years, **GABA** is a relatively new discovery in the field of neuroscience. It was not until the mid-twentieth century that scientists discovered the important role that GABA plays in the central nervous system. Today, many modern medications for anxiety, insomnia, and even epilepsy contain GABA. Additionally, we have a solid understanding of how regular levels of Magnesium and GABA can work together to produce a restful and productive night's sleep.

If you feel that you lack energy and passion for life, or if you feel that your health could improve, then start with your sleep. It is the most basic function our bodies perform, after all. And the best part is, sleeping requires no effort from you. All you have to do is find a dark room, a comfortable pillow, and let your body complete its natural repair function and hormone production. If you have trouble sleeping, you might try a Magnesium or GABA supplement to help your body relax and rest. You will be amazed at the results.

If you would like to purchase Magnesium supplements, please visit https://amzn.to/2lkKTm1.

If you would like to purchase GABA supplements, please visit https://amzn.to/2lj2nyV.

Chapter 2: Hydrate

"To keep the body in good health is a duty, for otherwise, we shall not be able to trim the lamp of wisdom, and keep our mind strong and clear. Water surrounds the lotus flower, but does not wet its petals."

-Buddha

Water is one of the most pervasive compounds on the planet. And yet, like many substances that are commonplace, people often take it for granted. The average adult's body is comprised of around 60 percent water, but instead of replenishing this valuable component to our bodies, we instead occupy our time drinking sugary sodas, coffee, juices containing high fructose corn syrup, and alcohol. People today just do not drink enough water. Many researchers estimate that the average person only consumes around two cups of water every day! This is just not enough to keep your body healthy and functioning at its peak.

Many ancient civilizations recognized the importance of water. For example, every known creation myth characterizes water as the origin of all life. In one of the Egyptian creation myths, the sun god is described as resting in an ocean before the beginning of the world. The Hindus also hold water as a sacred, life-giving symbol. Their holy books describe that every creature that exists on earth, even humans, emerged from the sea. Even today, they hold the Ganges River as sacred, and those who bathe in it can be purified from sin and other internal impurities. In the Judeo-Christian creation story, water is also a pervasive element. The water is never created but simply divided from the land and becomes the stage where the rest of creation occurs.

When people began to establish permanent civilizations, one of the main problems was creating a way to obtain drinkable water. One major archeological evidence we have of human's first attempts to gather drinkable water is the pervasiveness of wells across ancient sites—some of these wells dating to 2,000 BC. Ancient civilizations have also left behind other evidence of the importance of drinking water: aqueducts. The Romans, geniuses of technical engineering, created a plethora of aqueducts that ran throughout almost every corner of their empire. Water brought into cities by aqueducts helped provide the water supply for public baths, toilets, fountains, and even private homes. Some of these aqueducts were over 60 miles long. Likewise, in ancient Egypt, the people built complex networks of canals to bring water to themselves and their crops. To have created such extensive water systems demonstrates how important obtaining clean drinking water was for these ancient civilizations.

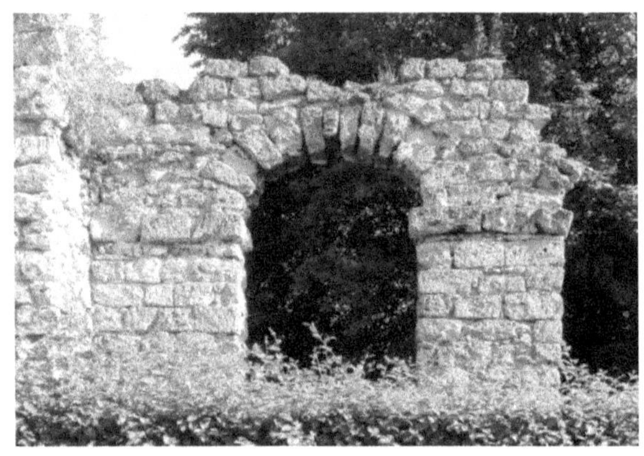

Water was not only needed to *maintain* health, but many ancient doctors and philosophers believed that drinking water could also *improve* one's health. Alcmeaon of Croton, an influential Greek doctor from the fifth century BC, was the first to observe a connection between the quality of drinking water and the overall health of a group of people. Many Greeks also believed that water had the ability to expel waste, impurities, and even illnesses from the body. In the writings of Hippocrates, another important Greek doctor, water was often described as a way to cleanse infectious wounds. In such cases, either seawater or rainwater would be prescribed, presumably because it would be the purest. In ancient Egypt, water was also important for healing. It was one of the main ingredients for almost all medications since many herbs and plants could be dissolved into water.

While many cultures used water as a basis for medicine, only a few used water as a medication all on its own. One example is the Desana tribe, a group of indigenous people from the Amazon rainforests. This civilization adopted the practice of praying over or singing to water before administering it to a sick person. The song helped to endow the water with what they called "intention" or specific healing instructions. The water would then act as a channel to carry the song or prayer directly to the afflicted area of the body. This practice still continues today within the Desana tribe and is starting to gain greater acceptance within some fields of medicine since the Japanese doctor Masaru Emoto discovered that the molecular structure of water can change based on different sound vibrations.

The people of ancient times knew how important water could be for both maintaining and improving overall health. But today, people often ignore the simple solution of increasing their daily intake of water. By simply drinking water more regularly, you can experience what our ancient ancestors did. If you adopt this one simple behavior, you can improve your health and happiness.

The most important thing that water does for your body is to act as a cleanser, flushing out the impurities in major organ groups as well as from individual cells. All of your body's major organ systems will work better when they are cleansed and properly hydrated. Just as in ancient times, water today is linked to detoxification and will help you purify every major system in your body.

Water is essential for brain health. Your brain, one of the body's most important organs, is made up of around 80 percent water. What's more, current research suggests that your brain cells require two times as much energy as other types of cells. Since water is one of the most effective ways to transport energy to your brain cells, by increasing your daily water intake you can increase your brain's functions. Your brain does not have its own way to store water, so the only way to keep your brain healthy and functioning is to adopt a habit of regular water consumption. Not only can water provide your brain with energy, but it also helps flush out harmful substances such as pollutants, toxic metals, and even radiation that are carried to the brain through your blood supply. Water can also deliver important nutrients to the brain to keep it functioning in top shape. By drinking water, you will be able to have a clearer memory and increased problem-solving skills, and even to reduce attention deficiency. There is nothing to lose but everything to gain if you increase your daily drinking water.

In addition to improving your brain's functions, water can also help your skin stay healthy and young. Water can help your skin achieve its needed moisture, which will keep it looking young and radiant. It is also important for bringing essential nutrients to the cells in your skin. By increasing the amount of water you drink daily, you can also reduce the skin's redness and puffiness. Additionally, water makes the skin firmer and will help prevent wrinkles. Without enough water, your skin will begin to prematurely age, developing more and permanent wrinkles.

Water also has the power to decrease some of the symptoms of inflammation, especially in joints. Water helps lubricate your body's joints, and if you are not drinking enough water, then there will not be enough water in your body to help your joints glide easily over one another. In addition, water will help you regulate your digestion. By staying hydrated, you will pass waste more regularly.

When your body is fighting off an illness, it is also important to drink water. When you have a cold, your body is trying its best to fight off harmful substances in your body. By drinking water, you will be providing fuel to your cells to continue the fight. Drinking water will also help you expel more mucus—an essential part of your body's cold-fighting powers. If you have a fever, continuing to drink water will also provide your cells with the fluid they need to stay strong and rid your body of the disease.

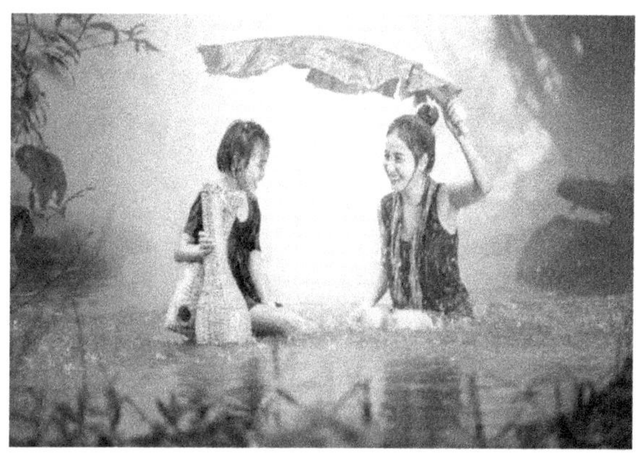

While the amount of water you consume daily will change depending on your level of activity, the weather, and your body weight, current medical doctors recommend that the average adult drink eight 8-ounce glasses of water every day. Following this recommendation will ensure that you are getting at least the minimum amount of water to avoid dehydration. If you want to increase your daily water intake, or you want a water intake regulated to your specific needs, you may want to try drinking half of your body weight in ounces. For example, if you weighed 150 pounds, then you should drink 75 ounces of water every day. That is more than the recommended 64 ounces daily. If you participate in sports, exercise, or spend a lot of time outside in the sun, you will also want to increase your daily water intake.

Even though people might know the many benefits the body receives from drinking more water, it can still be difficult to create a strong water-drinking habit. But, establishing this habit is essential for enjoying water's many health benefits. One of the best ways to drink more water is to drink water at certain times of the day. This more than anything else will help you establish a better water-drinking habit. Furthermore, the best time to drink water is first thing in the morning. If you drink water right when you wake up, before eating or drinking anything else, it will help to kick-start your body's natural detoxification process. It is also a gentle signal to your body that it is time to start the day, which includes starting your metabolism and increasing blood flow throughout your body. Next, you should drink water before meals. Establishing this habit will ensure that you are drinking a minimum of three glasses of water per day. Drinking water before a meal has also been shown to decrease the number of calories you consume at that meal, leading to weight loss and helping you to avoid overeating. You can also switch out other drinks during the day, such as coffee or soda, with a glass of water instead. This will help you increase the amount of water you drink, as well as decrease your daily sugar intake. Many people also find it helpful to set a timer at specific times during the day and to drink water at those times.

Sometimes the flavor or temperature of the water can prevent you from getting your daily hydration. If you find drinking water boring, you can add sliced fruit to your water to give it some flavor. Try to avoid artificial flavor mixes or drops, though, as these can contain preservatives and sugars that might counteract the benefits received from drinking pure water. It's also important that you drink water at a temperature you find comfortable. If you enjoy drinking ice-cold water, make sure that you always have enough ice in your freezer throughout the day and a water bottle that can maintain a cold temperature. Some people also enjoy drinking water that is room temperature or merely cool. This is also okay. If you drink water at an enjoyable temperature, then you are more likely to meet your daily water goals.

If you struggle to drink the recommended amount of daily water, increasing your <u>Vitamin C</u> can also provide you with many of the same benefits. Vitamin C, or ascorbic acid, is one of the 12 essential vitamins that humans need to survive. Generally, the body needs Vitamin C to develop and repair all types of tissue found in the body, which ultimately helps the body heal from wounds and recover from illnesses. Unlike many animals, humans cannot naturally produce vitamin C on their own. Instead, the only way to obtain this important vitamin is through a person's diet. But, like most nutrients the human body needs, most people are not getting enough Vitamin C through diet alone and are missing out on many of Vitamin C's special powers.

Similar to the benefits associated with drinking more water, increasing your daily Vitamin C intake, will give your body a boost against illnesses and toxins. Vitamin C will help protect you against free radicals and other toxic chemicals which could eventually lead to cardiovascular disease, cancer, or arthritis.

While we now know that a simple increase in Vitamin C will not *cure* the common cold, it can help the body fight against further complications. For example, by taking Vitamin C while experiencing a cold, you will prevent your body from experiencing pneumonia or further infections in the lungs. This vitamin contains important antioxidants that will give your immune system a natural boost. Vitamin C has also been found to be especially helpful to people who get sick regularly due to large amounts of stress.

Another one of Vitamin C's main roles is to function as an antihistamine. In other words, Vitamin C can help reduce inflammation and swelling during an allergic reaction or rash. This, in turn, can help improve the quality of your skin. Like water, Vitamin C can help your skin appear younger and prevent wrinkles. By increasing your daily dose of Vitamin C, your skin will be less dry, red, and will wrinkle less easily.

In addition to Vitamin C, <u>Aloe Vera</u> is another important substance that can help you stay hydrated. You'll probably recognize Aloe Vera as the sticky substance that you apply to your body after a sunburn. But, this plant has a lot more power than merely treating burned skin. If you take Aloe Vera internally, you can experience many benefits.

Aloe Vera is an ancient secret, with written evidence of this magical plant as far back as ancient Egypt, Greece, and India. There, Aloe Vera was considered the "plant of eternity" because all the antioxidants and vitamins that it contains help protect skin from aging. Most importantly, Aloe Vera helps prevent against damage from UV radiation and can even treat existing damage caused by UV radiation. This plant is also full of nutrients, including Vitamin C, folic acid, calcium, magnesium, and even potassium. With such nutrients, your body will be better prepared to fight off diseases and stay healthy. In the ancient world, the benefits of Aloe Vera were widely known. In fact, the army of Alexander the Great used Aloe Vera both externally and internally. They administered Aloe Vera to their wounds to prevent infection and speed up the body's natural healing abilities. Alexander's army also drank Aloe Vera juice to prevent infection in their bodies. This simple plant was said to have made the armies of Alexander unconquerable. In ancient India, the plant was nicknamed "oil of girls" because of its anti-aging properties. Although from the ancient world, these benefits can still be enjoyed today.

If you want to enjoy more energy, improve your body's immune system, and appear younger, simply increase your daily hydration. Whether that comes from drinking more water, taking a Vitamin C supplement, or enjoying the ancient benefits of Aloe Vera juice, you are sure to find energy and rejuvenation in hydration.

If you would like to purchase Vitamin C supplements, please visit https://amzn.to/2limY6x.

If you would like to purchase Aloe Vera supplements, please visit https://amzn.to/2lhYydg.

Chapter 3: Eat

*"Let food by thy
medicine and medicine
be thy food."*

-Hippocrates

The ability to find food and nourish the body has driven human existence for thousands of years. Since our bodies cannot naturally produce all the essential nutrients we need to live, eating is essential to living a healthy life. However, the way that we eat now is not always nutritionally adequate or beneficial and does not produce the same life-giving effects that humans enjoyed thousands of years ago.

Primitive humans expended a great deal of energy daily, because of the harsh physical demands on the body. These demands included finding food, hiding from predators, and enduring unpredictable weather patterns. Yet, despite these difficult living conditions, our ancestors were able not only to survive but to thrive. How could they accomplish such a difficult task?

It is widely known that our common ancestors, who occupied this planet nearly 10,000 years ago, were made up of nomadic tribes that survived through foraging for fruits, vegetables, grains and wild cereals, as well as hunting for meat. Many historians believe that hunting and eating meat are key to our ancestors' ability to survive such severe circumstances. Eating meat would give our ancestors a larger caloric intake and provide the necessary strength to survive. However, eating meat is not *the* answer. While meat did make up a part of these people's diet, their main source of energy came from pure complex carbohydrates and foods with low a low glycemic index, or slowly digestible sugars. Their diets were based on ancient grains and unrefined sugars because meat could only be found seasonally. And when meat was available, our ancestors did not always have great success in bringing home what they killed. Most early people obtained over 70 percent of their yearly calories from plants, including whole grains, fruits, and roots.

As societies evolved, they slowly began to stop hunting and gathering, and instead, began to farm, domesticate animals, and develop methods for preserving food during low-food production seasons. While farming allowed early humans to enjoy more leisure time, it ultimately reduced their nutrition. By farming and raising domestic animals, humans limited the amount of variety in their diet, leading to nutrient deficiencies and shorter life spans. Each population was also limited by geographical boundaries, and wherever in the world, a group decided to settle played a large role in determining the evolution of their dietary habits and future health.

In Northern Europe and the Scandinavian region, the ancestral region for many people currently living in North America, the people adapted to survive in their geographical location. For example, Northern Europe had harsh winters and short summers, which meant that they had a short growing season. So, instead of growing crops, many Europeans learned how to breed and domesticate animals that could more easily survive through the winter. Meat quickly became a staple of the European diet and was the source from which most nutrients were derived on a daily basis. Also, because of the harsh winters, learning how to preserve food was essential for survival. One of the staples of people's diet in this region was smoked or dried meats. In addition to meat, northern Europeans also learned how to preserve other foods. Some of the main foods they consumed and learned how to preserve were dairy products. Northern Europeans learned to make cheese, cultured or fermented milks, and butter, and consumed a lot of dairy products. The long winters also ensured that fresh fruits and vegetables were not always available, and when they were, it was usually for only a few months out of the year. To preserve the fruits and vegetables, the people also dried them or used sugar or salt to dehydrate them for the winter. While the northern European diet was high in protein, because of their preservation methods, it was also very high in sodium. Further, the high prevalence of dairy products from domesticated livestock led to increased amounts of saturated fats in their diet, resulting in cardiovascular diseases and weight gain.

On the other side of the continent, in Southern Europe and near the Mediterranean Sea, diets developed quite a bit differently. In ancient Greece, for example, cereals and grains made up a large part of people's nutrition. Unlike the "barbarians" in the north, Greeks had long summers and a large harvest. They spent a lot of time growing grains and living off of fruits and vegetables, especially olives. People in ancient Greece also chose not to eat much by way of red meats. The Greeks believed that tending domestic animals did not require much work since all one had to do was let the cow graze in a field. Because of this, eating red meats was considered shameful. Their diet was largely based on wines, grains, fresh fruits, and vegetables as well as olive oil, and is now considered one of the most healthful ways to eat. You can replicate the diet of the ancient Greeks by following a few essential steps. First, replace red meats with plant-based foods including vegetables and fruit as well as ancient grains and legumes. You should also replace the butter and creams of the northern European diet with healthy oils, such as olive oil. These simple tips can help you to enjoy your food better today.

In the ancient world, a person's economic status also played a huge role in determining diet and health. In ancient Rome, the wealthy often consumed meat products, and having meat on the table was considered a symbol of status and wealth. The poor, on the other hand, did not have the luxury to afford red meats. One example of this is the gladiator soldiers. Unlike the rich Romans who consumed red meats daily, the gladiator soldiers were only allowed the humblest of food. This included ancient wheat, small amounts of fish, and legumes. This strict diet led to many people in the ancient world calling gladiators "Barley Men" since ancient wheat made up such a large part of their diet. Animal protein was just not a part of these men's diet. And yet, they were able to become strong, highly capable warriors. We can learn from the diet of these poor men. By increasing our daily intake of simple, ancient wheat, we, too, can decrease our body fat and increase our strength.

The ancient wheat of the gladiators also supplied them with plenty of fiber. Dietary fiber, which is most commonly found in whole and unrefined grains, is an important part of maintaining digestive health. Fiber can also act as a detoxifier by helping your body to naturally expel harmful and unwanted substances. Soluble fibers can actually soak up harmful substances in your dietary track and help your body expel them. Eating a diet high in fiber can help you maintain healthy bowel movements as well as prevent harmful bowel-related diseases, such as hemorrhoids or diverticular disease. Overall, fiber can help encourage your body to produce healthier gut bacteria, which will improve your health overall. By adopting some of the eating practices of ancient gladiators, you can also enjoy the benefits of a diet high in fiber.

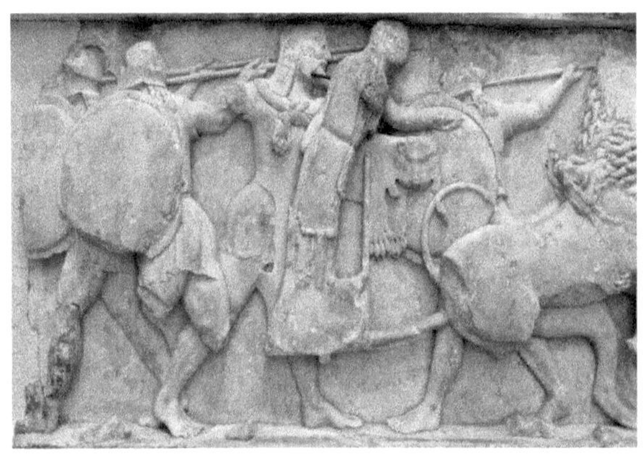

Additionally, the gladiators' high-fiber diet also helped gladiators to maintain healthy weights. Since fiber tends to fill you up faster, eating more fiber can help you feel full and stay full longer, ultimately avoiding the trap of over-eating and gaining weight. If you examine the ancient artistic depictions of gladiators, you will see that these men have very little abdominal fat and are often portrayed with clearly defined abdominal and chest muscles. Eating a diet of ancient wheat clearly helped gladiators stay lean.

Not only is fiber essential for maintaining a healthy body weight, but it can also help you control cholesterol and high blood sugar. Soluble fibers can absorb the excessive sugars in your blood and help remove it from your body, promoting healthy blood sugar levels. The fibers found in beans, oats, and bran can also help reduce low-density lipoproteins, or "bad" cholesterol, in your diet. Fiber also helps your heart by reducing blood pressure and decreasing inflammation. It's to your benefit to increase your daily fiber intake.

Currently, however, less than 50 percent of people living in North America consume the recommended daily fiber. Asians surprisingly consume about three times the amount of fiber that Americans do. Why are North Americans currently so fiber-deficient, while Asians enjoy a fiber-rich diet? Again, the answer goes back to how geography influenced dietary habits.

North Americans mainly come from Northern European descent, whose ancient diet was high in red meats, dairy products, and preserved foods. In Asia, especially regions of what is now China, the weather and climate were ideal for growing grains and cereals. In fact, archeological evidence supports China's long agricultural history. On the banks of the Yellow River, archeologists discovered preserved noodles, over 4,000 years old, which were made from locally grown grains including foxtail millet and broomcorn millet. Both of these grains are included in what is known in

Chinese culture as the "Five Grains." These grains include soybeans, hemp, foxtail millet, and broomcorn millet. These five grains have been a part of Asian diets for thousands of years and continue to provide a basis for Asian diets today. Because the people who settled in Asia had a lot of arable lands that could provide a variety of grains and cereals, they did not need to rely as heavily on meats or preserved foods to survive. Because of this, the Asian diet developed in a drastically different way from that of Northern and Southern Europe.

In addition to a rich variety of grains, ancient Asians also regularly ate fruits and vegetables including peaches, plums, and melons, as well as bamboo shoots and taro roots. These fruits and vegetables provided variety to the ancient Asian diet and also ensured that the people would receive the basic nutrients, vitamins, and antioxidants to keep them healthy and strong. Seafood also made up a large part of the Asian diet; fish, shellfish, squid, and even turtles were all consumed by ancient Asian people. Because they consumed so much seafood, their diets were high in <u>Omega-3</u>. This nutrient is essential to our diet because it helps encourage brain health and also prevents the effects of aging, such as arthritis and high blood pressure.

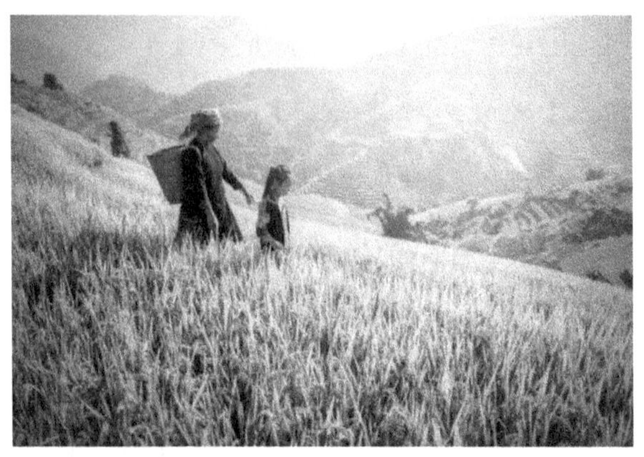

Ancient people received a lot of their Omega-3 from fish and seafood as well as soy products and certain nuts. While you could eat more fish to increase your daily intake of this vital nutrient, today's fish contain much higher levels of toxins and contaminants than the fish of thousands of years ago.

Many fish contain mercury, which can be detrimental to your health. Other foods high in Omega-3 are also high in calories and can lead to weight gain and heart problems later on in life. Therefore, if you want to receive the benefits of Omega-3 without the risks, supplements that contain Omega-3 are the best option.

Chinese diets were also strongly influenced by religion and philosophy. In about 500 BC, the philosopher Lao Tzu introduced new Taoist ideas to the Chinese people. These included ideas about medicine as well as food and the relationship between the two. In traditional Chinese medicine, food is considered to be the foundation for good health. Additionally, spiritual and physical health was deeply connected. Taoist philosophers, including Lao Tzu, believed that all foods can be divided into two groups: Yin and Yang. Maintaining a healthy diet included eating balanced meals that included both Yin and Yang foods. The ancient Chinese people believed that if you did not eat a balanced amount of Yin and Yang foods, you could become very sick. In general, Yin foods are the foods that grow on trees up in the air. Many fruits fit this category as well as soy-based foods, and many vegetables. Yin foods are categorized as "cool" foods and often help to hydrate the body. Yang foods, on the other hand, are known as "warm" foods and help dry out the body. They include foods that grow underground, such as onions, garlic, and ginger. Yang foods also include many types of meat and cheeses. Grains, such as rice or wheat, occupied a space in the middle and were seen as neither Yin nor Yang, but a little of both. By eating food from each of these categories during a meal, the Chinese people ensured that they were getting a healthy balanced meal.

Eating is not only essential for getting required nutrients for the body, but eating can also play a major role in how you emotionally feel and even the attitude you have towards life. The gladiators' diet and the diet of the ancient Chinese were rich in both Omega-3 and fiber. Both of these nutrients have been linked to helping your body not only be healthier but helping you feel better as well. For example, Omega-3 has been associated with helping people fight depression and anxiety as well as reducing many of the symptoms of these mental disorders. When you consume Omega-3, you are less likely to experience bouts of sadness and lethargy. You will also be less prone to worry or get nervous if you suffer from those symptoms already. This essential nutrient also helps enhance your brain cell receptors' ability to understand your surroundings and make wise choices. If your body is deficient in Omega-3, you will have a harder time making decisions that will lead to long-term happiness. Omega-3 is also essential for healthy eyes and vision. This nutrient is an essential part of the retina structure. By consuming more of it, you can prevent macular degeneration and improve the overall quality of your vision. When you can physically see clearly, it is easier to maintain a clear outlook on life and a positive attitude.

Fiber can also influence your attitude. Because fiber helps promote stabilized blood sugar levels, if you eat enough fiber, you can avoid feeling lethargic or unmotivated—two symptoms brought about by high blood sugar. Having high blood sugar can also make you become irritated and angry more quickly. Eating fiber can help you maintain a calm, relaxed attitude and avoid lashing out at those around you.

Eating is essential for life and helps provide the body with all the nutrients it needs to grow, fight diseases, and prevent illness. It's important to understand the origin of food and diet so that you know why you eat what you eat and how you can improve upon your current diet. Our ancient ancestors were limited in what they could eat based on where they settled and the geography and climate of the landscape. However, today, you have the opportunity to enjoy the advice and wisdom from all cultures. By making simple changes to the way you eat and think about food, you can drastically increase your health and promote an illness-free life.

If you would like to purchase Omega 3 supplements, please visit https://amzn.to/2M70z7D.

Chapter 4: Fast

"Instead of using medicine, better fast today."

-*Plutarch*

When you hear the word "fasting" you probably think of someone like Gandhi or Jesus, enlightened individuals who practice fasting as a way to experience spiritual illumination. While this can be one important benefit, fasting can also help your physical body to prevent disease and heal from illness, as well as maintain its weight.

Fasting, put simply, is the practice of abstaining from food for a period of time. This period could fluctuate anywhere from 12 hours to 21 days. At first, it might seem difficult to consciously fast. Food is an important part of our daily routines—it helps us measure the day into different parts and can play a large role in how we socialize and interact with people. However, each of us fasts every day. Between meals and during the night we pass hours without consuming food or nutrients. By increasing the intervals you spend between meals or consciously deciding to participate in the practice of fasting, you will see an improvement in both your body and your mind.

Fasting is not a new practice. People have been fasting since they first began to eat. Our hunter and gatherer ancestors fasted out of necessity since food was not always widely available. Unlike today, they were rarely able to eat three meals on an average day. As societies developed agricultural practices, fasting daily became less necessary because food was more readily available and could be preserved for use during less fruitful times. However, even in these societies, many people would still fast for long intervals between each meal, often not eating the first meal until 10 or 11 in the morning, and then only eating about two meals every day. Only wealthy people would eat more than two meals, but they also experienced obesity and other weight-related diseases.

Today, people tend to eat too often, and they do not fast hardly at all. This leads to a lifestyle where their stomachs and digestive tracts are always full and never have a break from working or the time to cleanse themselves. If you eat too often and do not fast regularly, your body will begin to store the extra nutrients, and this can lead to illness and disease. Eating too often can also dull your sensitivities and mind, causing you to make poor decisions. Fasting can truly help you live a richer, more satisfying life as well as experience optimal health.

Fasting has played a large role in many cultures and has been an important religious practice for thousands of years. Many religions including Buddhism, Hinduism, Christianity, Judaism, and Islam practice fasting as a part of their religious worship. In some of these traditions, fasting was only a religious practice and not necessarily connected with physical health. For example, the New Testament describes Jesus fasting for forty days. These forty days of fasting helped Jesus receive divine revelation and develop spiritual power. Today, many Christians follow this tradition established by Jesus by participating in Lent. Christians also fast when they want to experience a greater spiritual connection with God or receive spiritual revelations.

In general, fasting can help you to transcend your reliance on food and experience greater enlightenment. Whether you are spiritual or not, through fasting, you can experience a clearer mind and a greater awareness of your body's needs and desires. Since you no longer have to focus on physical hunger, you can instead focus on feeding and nourishing the mind and spirit. Fasting will also help you improve your senses, especially taste. If you are used to eating a lot of processed foods that are high in sugar and fat, abstaining from food for a period of time can help your body remove that addiction and can allow you to appreciate higher qualities of food.

In addition to spiritual benefits, some religions also emphasized the important role that fasting plays in health. In Buddhism, for example, fasting is a large part of the religious practice, but it is also part of a healthy lifestyle. In some of their religious books, Buddha encourages his followers to fast for one meal to fortify the body against illness. He is famously recorded saying, "When I do not eat the evening meal, I am more aware of my health, and I feel lightness, strength, and a sense of well-being." Many practicing Buddhist monks today do not eat after the noon meal. Other followers of Buddha will practice fasting less intensely, choosing only to fast during certain days or at times of meditation.

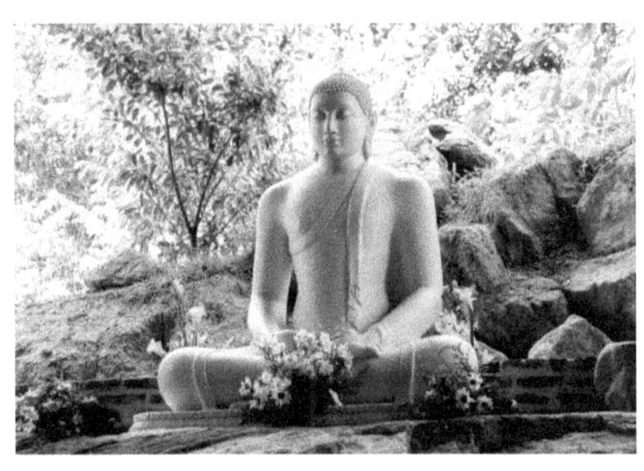

In ancient Greek culture, fasting was also closely associated with health. One of the first medical doctors, Hippocrates, said, "To eat when you are sick is to feed your sickness." In other words, ancient Greeks recognized the important benefit that fasting can have on a sick body. Fasting means

124

giving your body time to heal itself automatically and allowing your body the time it needs to naturally heal and recuperate. Hippocrates understood this important benefit of fasting and often prescribed fasting to his sick patients. Plato, a great Greek philosopher, also practiced fasting to increase both his mental and physical health. He is known to have said, "I fast for greater physical and mental efficiency." From his words, we see that Plato understood how important fasting was to the physical body as well as the mind and the spirit.

Taoism, a religion, and philosophy widely practiced in ancient China, also emphasizes the link between fasting and health. According to Traditional Chinese Medicine, diseases are mainly caused by eating food. Viruses, other germs, and toxins all enter the body because of something that was eaten. Therefore, to have a healthy body, a healthy diet is also needed. And the healthiest way to eat is to eat nothing at all so there will be no risk of contamination. An ancient Chinese parable says: "Those who eat meat are brave but cruel. Those who eat grain are smart but die early. Those who do not eat are immortal." By abstaining from food completely, followers of Taoism would be able to enjoy both the physical benefit of a long life as well as the spiritual benefit of immortality. For the common person, however, it is not recommended to abstain from food entirely. But, you can still enjoy the benefits of long-term fasting if you practice fasting in any capacity.

Similar to Traditional Chinese Medicine, Ayurvedic medicine from ancient India views the accumulation of toxins in the body and digestive system as the root of many of the body's diseases. Since fasting regularly allows the body time to cleanse from any accumulated toxins or harmful substances, it is the perfect practice to help your body heal from excessive waste and disease. Indian medicine encourages people to fast at least once a week to cleanse the body and purify the mind. It also sets aside certain days during the year, such as religious festivals, that should be dedicated to fasting and meditation.

One proponent of fasting was Gandhi, who fasted both for health and political reasons. Gandhi grew up in India during the British occupation. He watched for many years as his people and culture were oppressed by the British colonizers. Another problem Gandhi saw was that

Hindus and Muslims would not get along. To protest against the British occupation and encourage unity between these warring religious groups, Gandhi participated in over 15 long-term fasts during his life. Many of these fasts lasted for weeks, with the longest fasts lasting for 21 days. Gandhi had already fasted six other times, fasts that lasted anywhere from three to fourteen days, before embarking on his first fast to promote unity between the Hindus and Muslims living in India. This famous fast lasted 21 days. Although many people believed that Gandhi was starving himself, he was merely practicing the principles of the fast and allowing his mind and spirit control over his physical body. Also, despite Gandhi's rigorous fasts, he was able to stay alive and maintain his health.

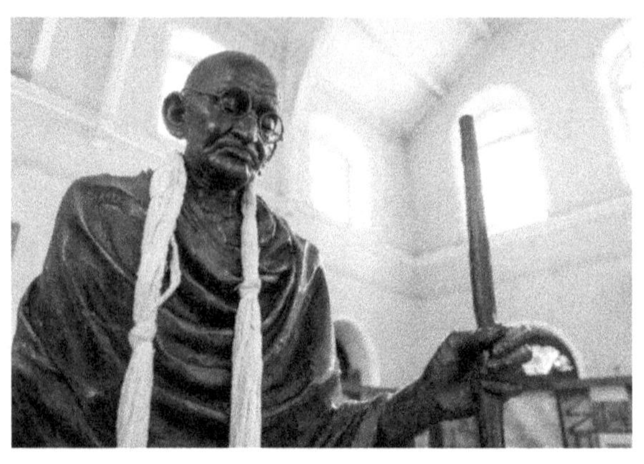

As you can see from the history, fasting has many benefits. One of the greatest benefits of fasting is its ability to naturally cleanse the body. By going without food, the body has the time it needs to dispel any toxins or waste and completely remove them. Because of this, fasting has enormous

132

benefits in maintaining a healthy digestive system. Fasting can help you reduce inflammation in your digestive tract. It can also prevent intestinal permeability, which is a condition where your digestive tract leaks excessive nutrients back into the bloodstream.

During a fast, however, you are not only cleaning out your digestive tract, but every cell in your body begins to detoxify. After going about 16 hours or more without food, your cells will begin a process called autophagy. This process is like a self-cleaning program that your cells adopt when they are not occupied with absorbing nutrients. During autophagy, your cells will release an enzyme that can remove the accumulated waste from inside the cell. Your cells also use this time to repair any damaged proteins and rebuild themselves. It is this process that is important for a long life and a youthful appearance.

Next, fasting is especially helpful in preventing illnesses from entering the body. For example, those who fast regularly are often protected from the harmful effects of cardiovascular disease and diabetes. Some people have even been able to reverse the effects of their diabetes through regular fasting. Fasting also helps to lower your blood pressure and promote healthy blood sugar levels. You can also sleep better on an empty stomach, and as this book has already discussed, sleep is one of the most important things you can do for your health.

Fasting can also help to increase your metabolism and can lead to burning more fat. After you have finished eating a meal, your body begins to digest your food—a process that can take up to three hours. At this time, your body will use different internal sources for energy. These sources include carbohydrates, fats, and proteins. Carbohydrates are the easiest for the body to break down, so they become the first source of energy. However, if you sustain your fast, your body will reach into its fat stores to provide itself with energy. Breaking down your fat stores is what gives your mind its clarity, a clarity that cannot be achieved except through fasting.

Fasting also helps you conserve energy. Every day, we spend a lot of time and energy obtaining food, preparing and cooking the food, and eating. Digestion is also a long process that requires a lot of energy from your body. Every system eventually needs a break, or it will become overworked. Through fasting, you can conserve the energy that is used when preparing, eating, and digesting your food. This, in turn, will allow you to have more energy for the things that matter, such as learning a new skill or spending time with people you love.

There are many different ways to fast, from increasing the time between meals to going without food for 24 hours or more. As with any new habit, it is important to listen to your body to know which method is best for you. Below are descriptions of a few ways to adopt the practice of fasting in your own life.

Time-Restricted Feeding. This fasting practice emphasizes the time of the day that eating occurs and how long you wait before eating again. It is based on the idea that our hunter and gatherer ancestors would only eat a few meals during the day and would rest at night. To practice this form of fasting, you should eat an early dinner, usually around four or five in the afternoon. Then you should not eat again for at least 16 hours.

If you ate dinner at five o'clock, then you would not break your fast until 8 AM the following morning. This type of fasting is very common, and you may already be practicing it without being aware. Also, this is a good type of fasting for those just beginning the practice. If you have never fasted before, try consciously abstaining from food between meals, and then slowly begin to lengthen the time spent between meals.

Intermittent Fasting. You can practice this type of fasting by abstaining from food for days at a time, usually no more than two days in a row. For example, you might not eat any meals on Monday and Tuesday, but from Wednesday to Sunday you would eat as you normally do. Usually, this kind of fasting is accompanied by either drinking water or juice. If you have never fasted before, try only fasting for 24 hours before moving on to something longer.

Periodic Fasting. This type of fasting is similar to intermittent fasting, except the goal is to fast for more than two days. Instead, those who practice this form of fasting try to fast anywhere from three to eight days. This type of fasting is usually accompanied by drinking water or juice. During this kind of fasting, many people will eat one small meal each day at the same time every day. You should not practice this type of fasting unless you are already well-practiced at other, shorter fasting intervals.

Water Fasting. You can practice water fasting for any period of time. During a water fast, you abstain from all food, including juices, but you are allowed to drink water. Many people will consume between three and four liters of water a day.

In addition to the fasting practices listed above, there are many more ways to fast. You can choose for how long, whether it is hours or days, and if you are going to consume any water or juice while fasting. However, above all, when fasting, it is paramount that you listen to your body and never try to fast for longer than you are physically able. Fasting has a lot of benefits, but these benefits can only be enjoyed if you are relaxed and your body is at peace. For example, fasting can help you be more alert and have a more positive mood, but if you are stressed out about eating or feelings of hunger, then fasting will only make you feel more anxious and can actually cause your body to reverse many of the health-promoting benefits of the practice. If you are new to fasting, try skipping just one meal, or lengthening the space of time between regular meals. You will begin to see the benefits of fasting in only a few days.

To learn more about fasting you can read *The No-Diet Diet-Intermittent Fasting Guide*. To purchase, please visit https://www.amazon.com/dp/B07DYYTZG3.

Chapter 5: Abstain

> *"The part can never be well unless the whole is well."*
>
> -Plato

Our modern diet has changed drastically from that of our ancient ancestors, and there are many substances we consume today that should not be a part of our diet at all. One of these harmful substances is refined sugar. Although not a drug, sugar has the potential to become an addictive substance, and sugar works to damage your body. It can also create illnesses and make you weak.

Everyone loves a good dose of sugar because it makes us feel good. But, if we really knew the far-reaching negative effects of what we were eating, we might not feel so good after all. Current research has linked eating large amounts of sugar to increased risks of numerous diseases, including diabetes, cardiovascular disease, and obesity. Eating too much sugar can also lead to increased inflammation and arthritis. Sugar naturally produces proteins and hormones that increase inflammation in the body. The toxins which sugar contains can also change the cellular structure of the cartilage—the soft cushioning between your bones—making it weaker and making your joints more prone to damage. Recent studies have even connected poor vision with an increased sugar intake. The consumption of a large amount of sugar leads to high blood sugar, a condition which causes the lens of the eye to swell. When this happens, it puts your eyes at a higher risk of developing cataracts, glaucoma, and it can even lead to the deterioration of your retinae, resulting in blindness. It's best to leave sugar off the table.

Additionally, eating sugar can also make you look old. When your body digests sugar, it breaks down the glucose which then attaches itself to proteins. Sooner or later, the glucose will attach itself to the proteins that are essential for creating smooth, firm skin—collagen and elastin. When this happens, it makes it more difficult for the proteins in your skin to repair, ultimately causing more wrinkles to appear quickly. Glucose can also suppress the human growth hormone. High levels of this hormone can help your body age more slowly, but if sugar is repressing its production, then you will age faster.

Sugar is also connected with increased illness. If you are eating too much sugar, your body will fill itself up on what are called "empty calories" or calories that contain no nutrients. This does not leave room in your body for vital nutrients such as vitamins, fiber, and protein. If you are not nourishing your body properly, it weakens your immune system, making it easier to contract an illness and even making it harder to recover. A study conducted by Ruslan Medzhitov, a Yale professor, revealed that glucose (most commonly found in sugar) can decrease your body's ability to fight a bacterial infection. Also, it is widely known that eating sugar can lead to an increased risk for diabetes and heart disease. As the sugar enters your bloodstream, your body produces insulin to balance the levels of sugar in your blood. If you consume more sugar, your body will produce more insulin which can eventually lead to insulin resistance, high blood sugar, weight gain, and diabetes.

As our world modernized, large food companies tended to add sugar to everything, to make it more appealing to buyers and especially to children. However, it was not always like this. When our ancestors ate the food they grew within their own communities, the problems associated with sugar appeared far less and were less widely spread. If you want to change your health, appear younger, and ultimately live a happier, longer life, you must avoid sugar.

Just because refined sugars and artificial sweeteners cause such harmful effects does not mean that you can never enjoy something sweet. Honey is a natural and safe alternative to many of the other modern sources of sugar. Unlike sugar, which only contains fructose and glucose, honey also contains water and digestive enzymes, as well as minerals such as Magnesium and Potassium. Additionally, since the bees have already added enzymes to the honey to help it break down, our body has to do less work when digesting honey. Finally, no one has ever gotten a cavity from eating honey, so it's safe for your teeth.

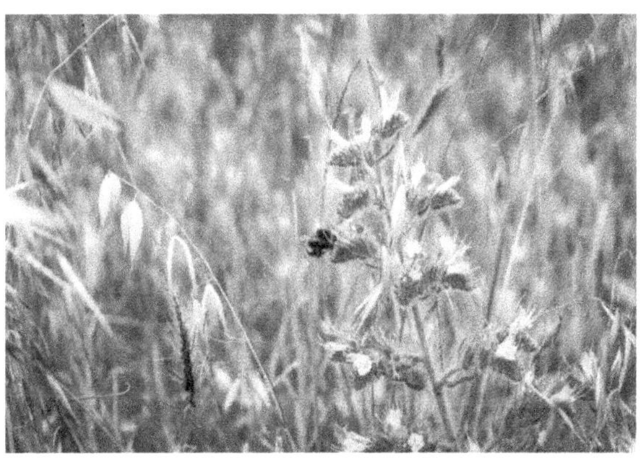

Ancient civilizations have long recognized the valuable product produced by bees, and evidence of this dates back to cave paintings found in Spain over six thousand years ago. The people from these ancient civilizations did not just use honey as a sweetener, but many people also used it as a form of medicine. In ancient Egypt, for example, almost all of their known medications—both digestible medicine and topical salves—contained honey in some form. Egyptians also used honey to reduce inflammation and swelling in the joints.

According to ancient Chinese medicine, honey had a

balanced character—meaning that it did not represent either Yin or Yang but fell somewhere in the middle. This made honey an ideal substance for medications to help the body become rebalanced. Ancient Chinese writings even mention that honey can be used to help an individual stay fit, as well as improve digestive health. From these examples of the past, we learn that honey is a much safer—and more useful—alternative to today's processed sugars.

Even young children know that sugar is bad for you, but many people are shocked to learn that milk is also harmful. For years, parents have taught their children that they needed the calcium from milk to grow big and strong. However, the truth is that cow's milk contains zero nutrients that you cannot obtain from more natural and sustainable sources. And what's more, drinking milk is an unnatural process that can lead to weight gain, an increased risk of diabetes, and even cancer.

One of the biggest arguments against drinking milk is that it's unnatural. Many people will argue that it is the most natural thing in the world since when we were first born, we drank milk. But that was milk produced by a human, tailored specifically for that growing infant. Although we drink our mother's milk as a child, it's completely unnatural to consume the milk of another mammal. No other animal will drink the milk of another animal like humans chose to do. You will not ever see an elephant drinking the milk of a giraffe, or a horse drinking the milk of a cow. So why would we drink milk other than from a human? Furthermore, all other mammals stop consuming milk after around the first year of their life. This is because the first year of an infant's life is the time in which it will experience the largest growth rate. For humans, a baby will increase its total weight by about 300 percent in the first year. A calf, on the other hand, increases its total body mass by over 1,500 percent in just the first year of its life. Not only do humans not need to consume human milk after their first year to maintain their rapid growth, they absolutely do not need to continue with a 1,500 percent growth increase that comes from drinking the milk of a cow.

Because milk is so high in protein and fat, it can also lead to weight gain. Drinking milk can quickly make you reach your daily calorie limit without even realizing it and thus lead to an increased caloric intake, ultimately causing you to gain weight. In fact, one of the number one recommended techniques for people trying to *gain* weight is to increase their milk consumption. Not only does the fat contained in milk add to your middle, but fat is a great solvent which quickly absorbs the many pesticides and chemicals used on the commercial land where dairy cows are raised. When you drink cow's milk, you are not only consuming the milk but also all those harmful chemicals used on the land. Cows are also treated with a smorgasbord of antibiotics and growth hormones. When you drink milk, you also absorb the antibodies and hormones used to unnaturally increase a cow's development. Exposure to such antibiotics, especially in young children, has been linked to increased risk for developing type 1 diabetes later in life. In short, there is nothing natural about our current milk consumption.

Milk also contains a lot of sugar in the form of lactose. Around 80 percent of people are intolerant of this type of sugar because it is not naturally produced in the body. That means that only 20 percent of the world's population has developed the enzyme needed to break lactose down into a digestible compound. Many researchers have traced the first milk drinkers to the region between the Balkans and Europe. But today, many people from Southern Europe and Asia cannot stomach milk.

In addition to being so unnatural and causing weight gain, many studies have shown that drinking milk can lead to increased risk of cancer. Recent studies suggest that consuming dairy products may lead to an increased risk for prostate cancer in men and an increased risk for breast and ovarian cancer in women. For example, in 2003 the Karolinska Institute—Sweden's leading medical institute—published a study that reported a link between a man's dairy consumption and his risk of prostate cancer as well as a woman's dairy consumption and her risk for breast cancer. Later studies built upon this link and proved that the negative effects of consuming dairy products as a child—especially milk—could be seen later in life in the development of these types of reproductive cancers. Another foundational study that linked drinking milk to cancer development was conducted by Dr. T. Collin Campbell. While doing research in India, Dr. Campbell noticed that children from rich families were often diagnosed with a rare form of liver cancer while the children from poorer families were not. After conducting more research, he concluded that the one cause for this cancer was the increased amount of animal proteins that the richer children had access to. One protein he tested, in particular, is called casein and it is most common in cow's milk. When these children had access to cow's milk, their cancer rapidly spread. However, without the milk, the carcinogen causing the liver cancer could not develop. All this research, both Dr. Campbell's and the studies produced by the Karolinska Institute, appear to reveal two things: first, that milk on its own can increase a person's risk for certain types of reproductive cancer, and second, drinking milk when another carcinogen is already present in someone's body can exacerbate the cancer's growth.

Even though you might be aware of all the negative side effects of drinking milk, it can still be hard to remove milk from your diet. Dairy products make up a huge part of the average person's diet, so learning to live without it can seem impossible. Luckily, there are many alternatives to help you make the switch. For example, nowadays it is quite easy to purchase milk from plant-based sources, such as almond milk, soy milk, or cashew milk. Each of these options is much healthier and is not associated with the negative health effects of cow's milk. The benefits to making the switch to plant-based milk can be seen in the average Asian's diet. Due to the way that nutrition and diet developed, many people in Asian countries do not consume nearly as much milk as people from the United States or Western Europe. Instead, their diet consists of whole grains, vegetables, tofu, and other soy products. Dairy products are largely absent. Because of this, people in Asia are generally healthier, are at reduced risks for breast cancer and prostate cancer, and often live much longer as well.

Another large part of the typical Asian diet is green tea. Many people are aware of the amazing health benefits of green tea, but fewer people know of green tea's stronger and better cousin: <u>Matcha Green Tea</u>. Matcha Green Tea contains all the same nutrients and health benefits of regular green tea but at a much more concentrated dose. But what makes Matcha better than regular green tea? Matcha translates as "powdered tea." While preparing traditional green tea, you infuse the hot water with the tea leaves but discard the leaves before drinking. With Matcha, the green tea leaves have been ground up into a fine powder, so you are getting about 10 servings of green tea with just one serving of Matcha Green Tea, along with all the nutrients green tea has to offer. Because you consume the entire tea leaf, Matcha Green Tea is also grown differently than regular green tea. During its last weeks, a shade cloth is placed over the Matcha tea plant so that the amount of chlorophyll will increase. Chlorophyll, the plant-based element that gives Matcha Green Tea its "green," is so important because it has the ability to detoxify your body by eliminating chemicals and heavy metals.

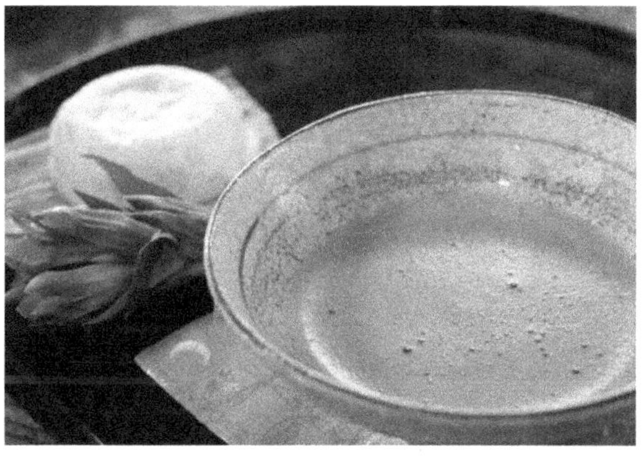

One of the primary benefits of drinking Matcha, however, is that it contains antioxidants in abundance. In total, Matcha contains over 6 times the amount of antioxidants as other "superfoods" including goji berries or blueberries. Antioxidants are an important part of a healthy diet, offering anti-aging benefits as well as preventing many chronic diseases including heart disease and cancer.

That's right, the antioxidants contained in Matcha Green Tea can also help you fight cancer. Matcha has a very unique group of antioxidants called catechins. This type of antioxidant cannot be found in other foods, but it has the amazing superpower of fighting cancer. Catechins help reverse the effects of free radicals from UV light and radiation that you experience every day. In sum, drinking Matcha Green Tea can help you reverse many of the negative effects brought about by drinking milk.

In ancient Japan, Matcha Green Tea was associated with meditation. Both the preparation and the drinking of this tea provided the focus for ancient

Japanese tea ceremonies. Consuming Matcha provided the drinker with the time to slow down and focus on the moment rather than the future or the past. You can replicate these same meditative practices in your own preparation and drinking of Matcha Green Tea.

To purchase your own Match Green Tea, please visit https://amzn.to/2lim6yP.

Chapter 6: Meditate

"As gold purified in a furnace loses its impurities and achieves its own true nature, the mind gets rid of the impurities of the attributes of delusion, attachment, and purity through meditation and attains reality."

-Adi Shankara

In the fast-paced world, many people struggle with the feelings and impacts of stress. It seems almost impossible to escape at times. Stress is also one of the main reasons people report on visiting doctors' offices, and there are many types of stress-related illnesses. One of the best ways to avoid stress in your life, and consequently avoid the many harmful side effects of stress, is to adopt a practice of daily meditation. Many experts recommend simply 20 minutes a day to help you experience optimal health benefits.

Meditation has been practiced by many ancient cultures. Most famously, we know that the eastern world, such as China and India, practiced meditation regularly—both as part of their religion and as a philosophical exercise. In ancient India, meditation has significance as both a religious and a cultural practice. The earliest written evidence of people engaging in meditation practices comes from a Hindu religious branch called Vendantism. Writings from this period make some of the first mentions of meditation and date back to 1500 BC. The written examples from China in the Taoist and Buddhist traditions date back to 500 BC—nearly 1,000 years later!

Many meditation practices in the Hindu tradition are done with a spiritual purpose in mind. Meditation helps one to achieve unity between their physical body and their eternal soul. In ancient

China, meditation served a similar purpose. Meditation was an essential part of the path towards reaching nirvana—or the ultimate enlightenment. In both ancient traditions, meditation practices combined intense mental focus with body postures, deep breathing, and sometimes visualization or mantra repetition.

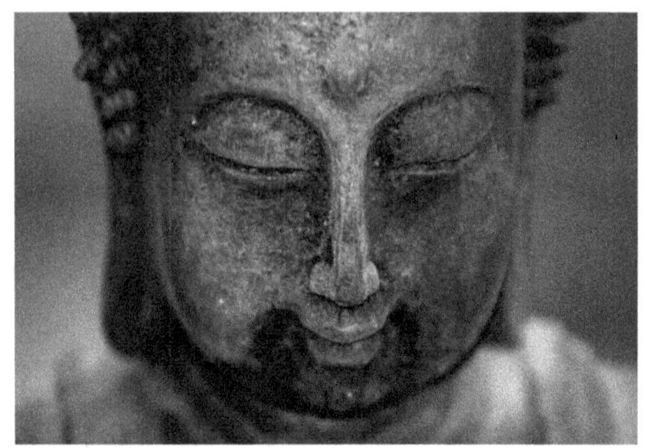

However, meditation is not just an eastern practice. Many ancient cultures from the west also practiced and taught meditation. For example, the ancient Greeks were devoted to the practice of meditation. In this culture, the word for meditate was "melete" which simply refers to a type of

182

disciplined study. "Melete" was also the name for one of the three muses that poets and artists would pray to for inspiration. In this sense, meditation for the ancient Greeks was a way to allow inspiration to flood the mind and to focus one's thinking on a singular activity. Additionally, the Oracle at Delphi is famously known to have said, "Know thyself." The oracle was the spiritual center of the ancient Greek's world, and it's telling that this spiritual advice is directed inward. Meditation would have most likely been required to reach this enlightened state. One of the popular Greek sages, Empedocles, also encouraged and taught meditation practices. He lived around 400 BC and taught his followers to search beneath their crowded, everyday thoughts to reach a higher reality. He also taught the importance of focused thinking to reach enlightenment.

In the Roman world, people also practiced meditation. One of the great spiritual leaders during the first century AD, Plotinus, was a proponent of focused thinking as a way to achieve self-understanding. He famously taught, "close your eyes and awaken to another way of seeing." Through his prescribed meditation practices, people in the ancient Roman world learned to relax the mind and body to find peace and understanding.

Meditation became more widely popular in the late 1960s and 70s when there was a resurgence of people interested in eastern medicine and health practices. Part of that resurgence movement was Dr. Herbert Benson, a medical doctor trained at Harvard. In 1971, Dr. Herbert Benson developed the revolutionary idea called "The Relaxation Response." After researching meditation for decades and examining the brains of Buddhist monks, Herbert Benson noted the difference in stress levels between those who practiced meditation and those who did not. In a nutshell, "The Relaxation

Response" is, in the words of Dr. Benson, "a physical state of deep rest." Entering into this rest can help your body change the way it reacts to and interacts with stress. Ultimately, it helps both your body and your mind to reach a point of total relaxation through traditional meditation practices.

Since his study, numerous other scientific research projects have been conducted on the physical and emotional benefits of daily meditation. Many of the benefits directly affect the mind.

For example, through meditation, you can increase your self-esteem and encourage self-acceptance. You will become a more optimistic person and will be more aware of your surroundings and your body's physical and emotional responses. Meditation can also help reduce the symptoms of depression and anxiety as well as help you feel less lonely. And, when you do engage in social interactions, they will become more engaged, because you will be more aware of the people around you and their needs.

With this increased sense of awareness, you will also reduce your impulsive decisions and worry less about the decisions you do make.

In addition to the many mental benefits of daily meditation, you will also experience huge amounts of positive physical responses. Most prominently, the deep sense of relaxation that accompanies meditation helps to lower your blood pressure. If you engage in meditation practices every day, you can help to encourage lower blood pressure on average in your body. Deep relaxation also encourages better blood circulation in your body. With lower blood pressure and improved circulation, you will also benefit from a reduced risk of cardiovascular disease.

Meditation directly taps into your central nervous system to promote healthy responses to stress. During meditation, you activate the parasympathetic nervous system. This is the part of the nervous system that is in charge of returning your body to relaxation and calm after experiencing high-stress situations or even physical danger. While this part of your nervous system is at work, your body will begin to repair and rebuild itself from any damage that it experienced during the stressful situation. Daily meditation will also help decrease inflammation in your body and can help improve the symptoms of asthma. Meditation truly allows your body the space and time it needs to rejuvenate naturally.

Daily meditation has also been shown to directly benefit the immune system. While in the deep relaxation stage of meditation, your body will decrease the production of a hormone called cortisol. This hormone is released when your body is stressed out or under a lot of pressure. While high levels of the cortisol hormone are in your body, your immune system has a slower response and is unable to fight diseases and illnesses the way it should. Daily meditation allows your body the time to rebalance your hormones and reduce the cortisol in your body. Overall, this will help your immune system function properly and will increase your healthy responses. Many scientific studies suggest that you can experience up to 50 percent less disease in your life by adopting simple meditation practices.

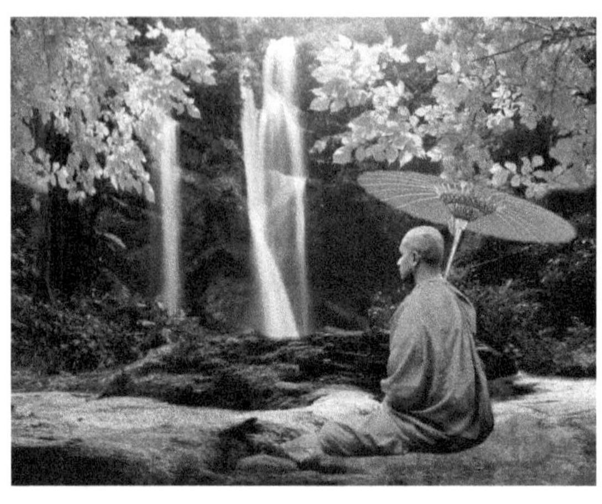

You can also promote healthy brain activity. In fact, while meditating, there is increased blood flow to different parts of your brain, specifically regions associated with memory and emotion. This means that through meditation, you can encourage positive thinking and will ultimately have a better outlook on life. With just a few minutes of meditation every day, you can create a positive attitude for yourself. Because meditation directly affects the part of your brain associated with memory, meditation can help you improve your short- and long-term memory. You will also experience improved creative thinking and problem-solving skills. Finally, because meditation trains your brain to be hyper-aware, you will be able to more easily ignore distractions and focus on the tasks at hand.

Meditating just before bed is also a healthy practice. Meditation can help you slow your breathing and reduce your heart rate, important physical responses that need to happen before you can enjoy a better quality of sleep. Since you receive so many benefits from sleeping, meditation before bed can help you gain all the health benefits of a good night's rest.

The benefits associated with meditation, including lower heart rates and blood pressure are also known to alleviate the symptoms of many serious medical problems and diseases such as arthritis, anxiety, infertility, hypertension, insomnia, depression, cancer, and ultimately aging. With all these benefits, there is no reason not to start meditating today!

However, in many people's busy schedules, it can be hard to find the time to dedicate yourself fully to meditation. It is also hard to maintain such intense focus for long periods of time. But, with a little work, you can find simple ways to meditate that will greatly increase your health. In fact, those who practice meditation for simply 20 minutes a day were able to see immense physical and mental improvements in just a few weeks.

One of the simplest ways to practice meditation is to engage your brain in intense focus while doing a mundane activity such as washing the dishes or walking. Encourage your brain to stay in the here and now. Try to stay focused and allow your thoughts to pass without judgment through your mind.

Additionally, the best time to meditate is in the morning or at night. These are the times when your body is already in a natural state of relaxation, and you will be able to enter a state of deep relaxation more quickly. Also, try to avoid meditating within two hours after any meal. If your digestive system is still working, it will be harder for your entire body to enter a state of deep relaxation.

If you want to attempt something a bit more intense, try the following:

1. Begin by finding a quiet room where you will undisturbed for the 10 to 20 minutes while you are meditation.

2. Sit in a comfortable position. This could be

cross-legged on the floor
or even in a chair.

3. Next, close your eyes.
Begin by focusing on your
breathing. Breathe in
through your nose and out
through your mouth. Do
not try to breathe at a
slower rate at first, since
your breathing will
naturally slow down as
your body becomes more
relaxed.

4. Focus on the muscles in
your body. Begin with the
muscles at your feet and
work your way up to the
top of your head.
Dedicate however much
time you need to make
sure that muscle group is
well relaxed before
moving on to the next
muscle group. Do not
forget to continue
focusing on your
breathing while

progressing through your muscle groups.

5. After you have completed this process and have given attention to every muscle group in your body, allow yourself to slowly become more aware of your surroundings. Notice the sounds around you. Try to interpret the smells you notice.

6. Slowly open your eyes again and observe what you see around you. Do not try to stand for a few minutes after you have finished this process. Just let yourself naturally come back to your body as your surroundings come into focus.

One important part of meditation is avoiding letting your mind wander. You must keep your mental attention focused on one thing. Because of this, many people who practice meditation will listen to guided meditation audio tracks. If you choose this method of listening to a prerecorded meditation audio, focus fully on each word and really try to live in the moment. You can also repeat a mantra or a sound over and over again to help your mind stay focused. Dr. Benson recommends a word that brings you happiness or creates a positive atmosphere such as "love" or "peace." If you are repeating a certain phrase, make sure that you speak in rhythm with your breathing. Also, if the word or sound you have chosen leads to negative thoughts of any kind, stop and choose another word.

If you feel that you are unsuccessful at your first attempt to meditate, do not become discouraged. Remember to maintain a positive attitude. Relaxation will come to your body when it is ready and prepared. If you make meditation a habit, you will be experiencing the positive effects of this practice in a few weeks.

To encourage your body's relaxation, you may also want to consider taking a <u>Neuro Nutrients</u> supplement. This supplement contains amino acids as well as B Vitamins and *Ginkgo biloba*—a plant with many magical properties, including treating high blood pressure, improving overall heart function, and even encouraging healthy brain functions. This unique combination of nutrients found in Neuro Nutrients helps promote a healthy nervous system and can also reduce stress-related fatigue and mental exhaustion. Additionally, Neuro Nutrients contains the important amino acid L-Tyrosine which is essential to the function of your body's immune system and help protect your skin from UV light. By taking this supplement, you will increase your immune system's abilities as well as preserve your skin from harmful radiation and wrinkles. This supplement in conjunction with daily meditation will help you to achieve these physical and mental benefits even faster.

If you want to learn more about meditation, you can read _The Ancient Secrets of the Fountain of Youth_ by Peter Kelder available at https://amzn.to/2JS63GM.

To purchase Neuro Nutrients, please visit https://amzn.to/2K09eYR.

Conclusion

Here at the close of *The Magical Secrets of Healing: Ancient Remedies and Diet Hacks with Mystical Age Reversing Properties*, we hope that you learned all you were able from the secrets of the past. Studying these secrets and adopting them into your life as daily practices will help you be healthy, heal from disease, live long, be fit, and experience joy. Remember that change at first can be hard work, but these practices are simple and have large rewards if you can follow through.

Learning from ancient civilizations and their philosophers is the best way to experience positive health benefits. Use the daily practices of sleeping, eating, and drinking to increase your body's potential to heal. Adopt ancient practices of meditation and fasting to promote natural healing and prevent disease. You will find success and happiness through these simple practices.

If these secrets were able to help you, leave a review on Amazon so that they can be shared with everyone. Good luck on your personal health journey!